Table of Contents

Hello Beautiful!

My name is Makenzee, and I am the proud founder of Spoonful of Happy.

Thank you from the bottom of my heart for taking time out of your busy

schedule to view the content I have worked so hard to provide for you.

Without you, none of this would be possible! I am truly living a dream.

 At Spoonful of Happy, we have proudly dedicated ourselves to promoting

healthy living from the inside out. But we also understand how much fun it can

be to experiment with beauty products! Since our skin is the largest organ in

our bodies, it is only fair we give it some love and attention too.

Spoonful of Happy is in the process of creating more books with high quality

content. This is the first of many books to be released for our followers!

Enjoy!

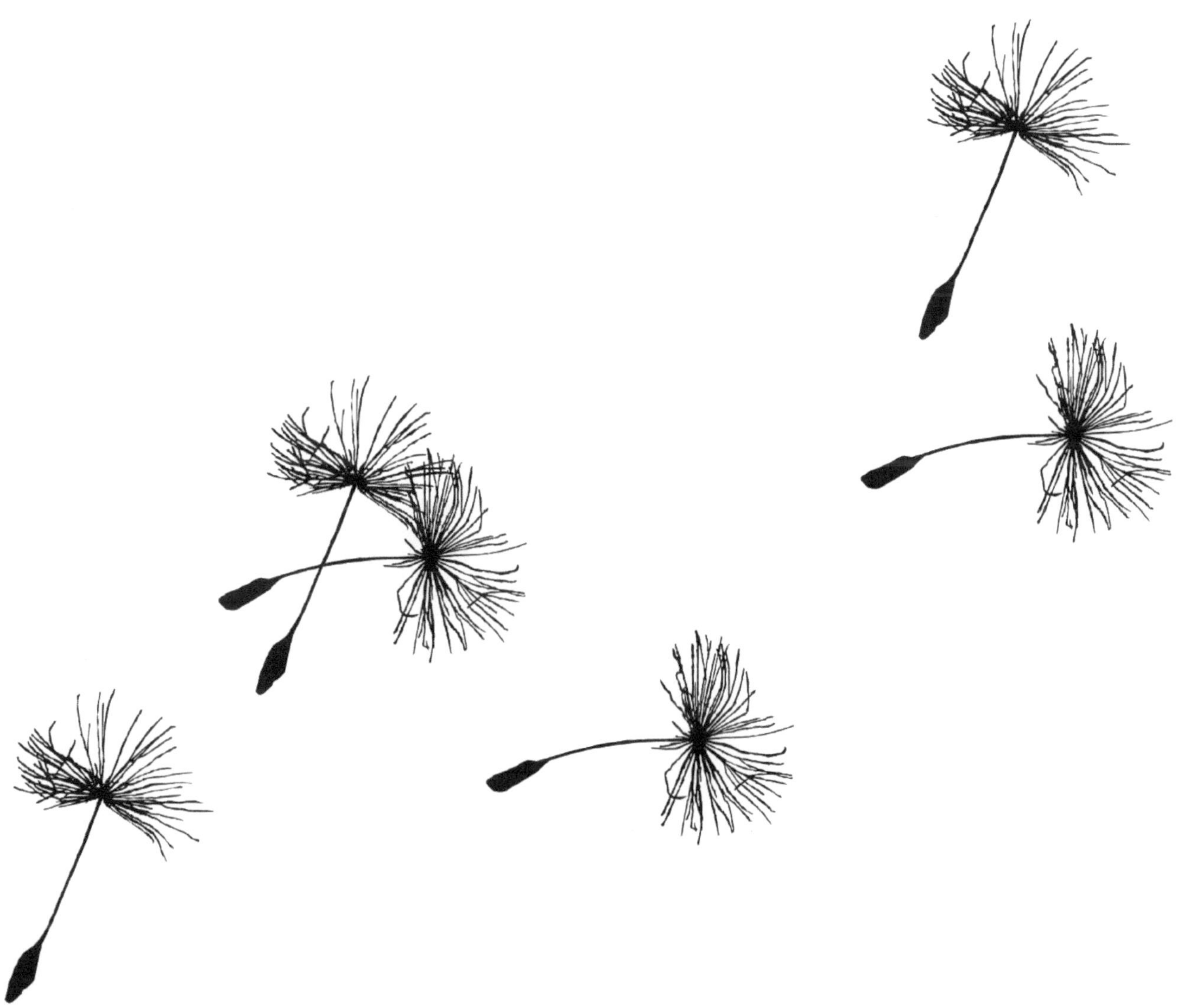

Time to Get Started!

Whether it is a girls' night in, bachelorette weekend, or a night off alone with your dog… there are not many scenarios where this book will not provide entertainment and come in handy.

 The hustle and bustle of living a busy life makes it easy to neglect our self-care. We are ALL guilty of it. Now is the time to kick off your shoes, and pour yourself a glass of wine! In the palm of your hands you have a book full of fun and natural skin care recipes to try. Practicing self-care can be challenging, but why not start showing yourself some love starting with this book? The amount of joy a healthy and balanced life can bring is limitless!

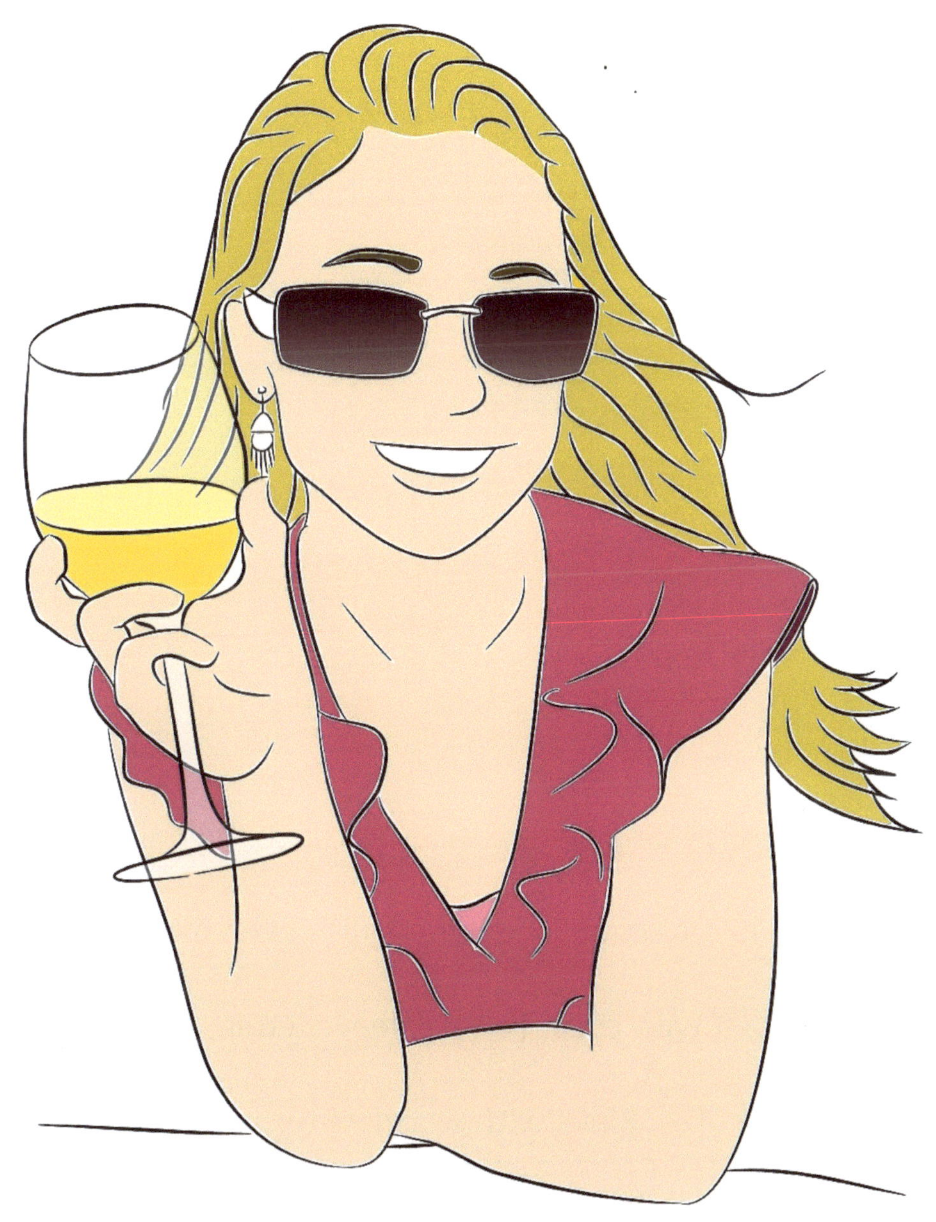

Lemon Blackhead Slayer

Helps remove dirt from pores, difficult blackheads, and assists in preventing future breakouts.

Ingredients:

- 1-2 Egg Whites (preferably organic)

- 1-2 tsp Fresh Lemon Juice

Instructions:

Beat egg white(s) well. Add fresh lemon juice. Stir.

I would <u>not</u> recommend adding any extra lemon juice. If your skin is extremely sensitive, use 2 egg white to dilute the lemon juice even more. Apply mixture to clean face, avoid contact with eyes. This will leave a thin, shiny film. Allow face mask to sit for 10-12 minutes. Rinse with warm water, pat dry with clean towel.

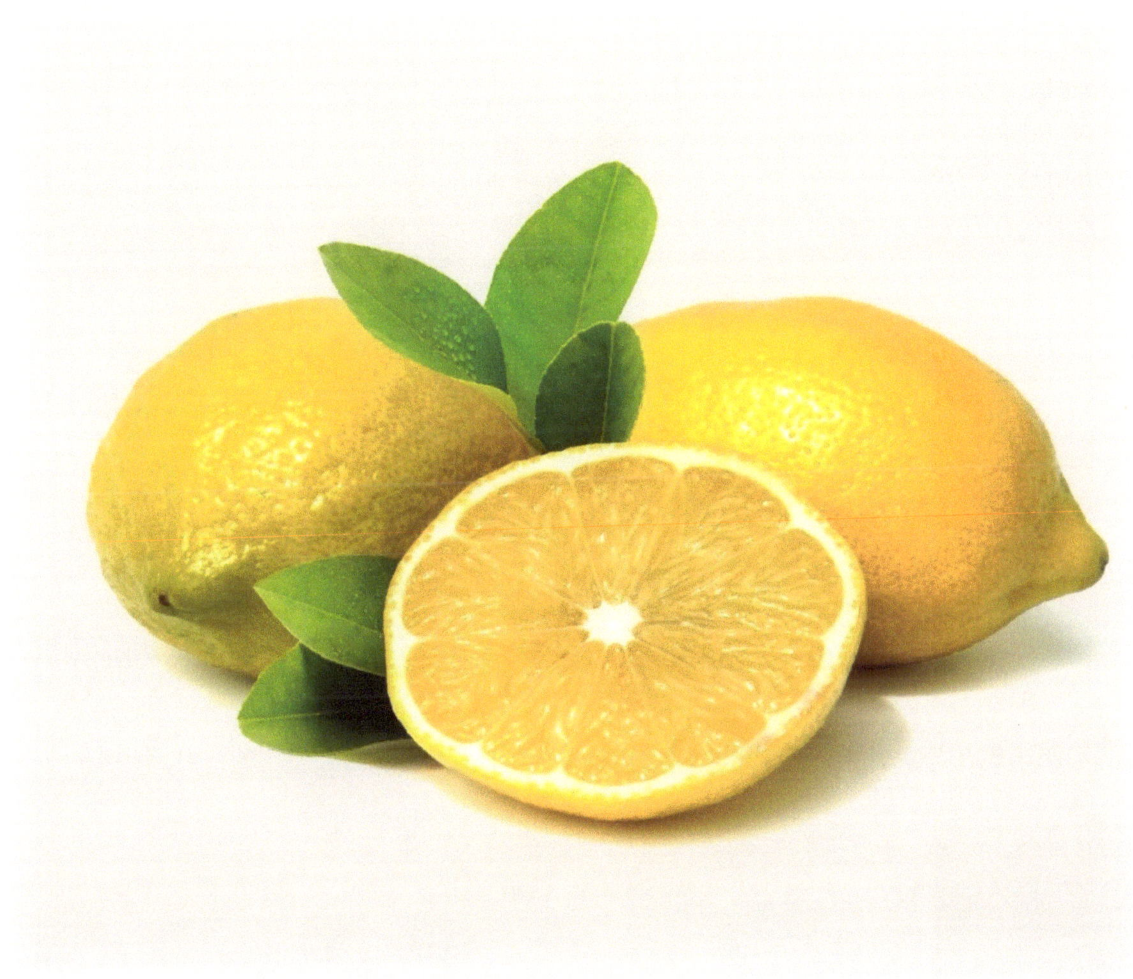

Avocado Oasis

Extremely hydrating, cool and refreshing, controls redness, provides natural glow.

Ingredients:

- ½ Ripe Avacado

- ½ Ripe Banana (the riper, the better!)

- 1 Tbsp. Olive Oil

Instructions:

Mush avocado and peeled banana together. Stir in olive oil. Apply liberally to clean skin. Let mask sit for 15-20 minutes. Rinse with warm water, pat dry with clean towel.

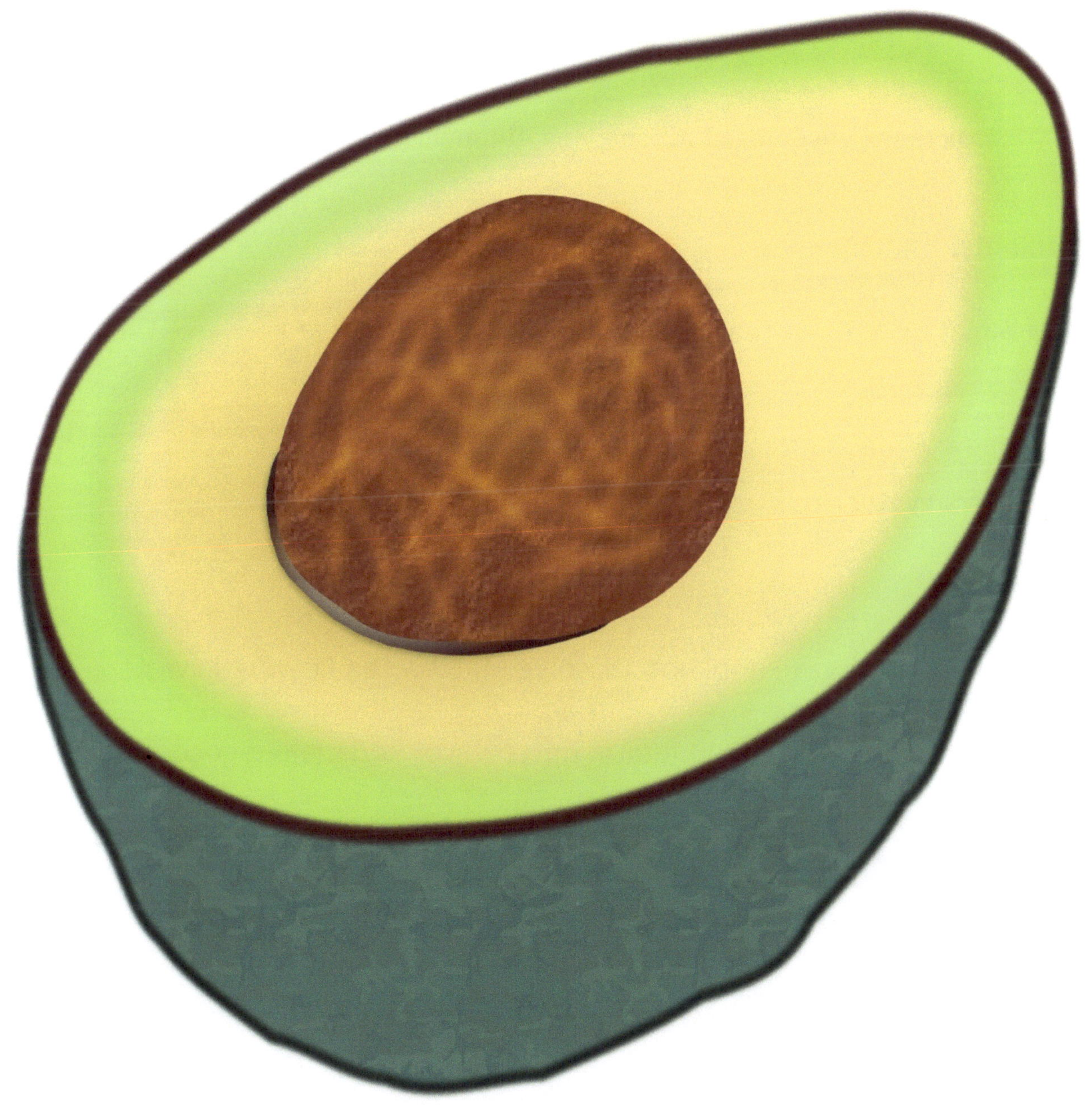

Matcha Redness Eraser

Assists with evening skin tone, and eliminating troubling redness.

Ingredients:

- 1 tsp. Raw Matcha Tea Powder

- 1 tsp. Coconut Oil

- 1 Tbsp. Water

Instructions:

Heat water in microwave until hot. Dissolve Matcha Tea Powder in water

stirring thoroughly. Melt coconut oil in microwave. Add melted coconut oil to

Matcha Tea and water mixture. Stir until well blended. Apply to clean face.

Allow to sit for 10-12 minutes. Rinse with warm water, pat dry with clean towel.

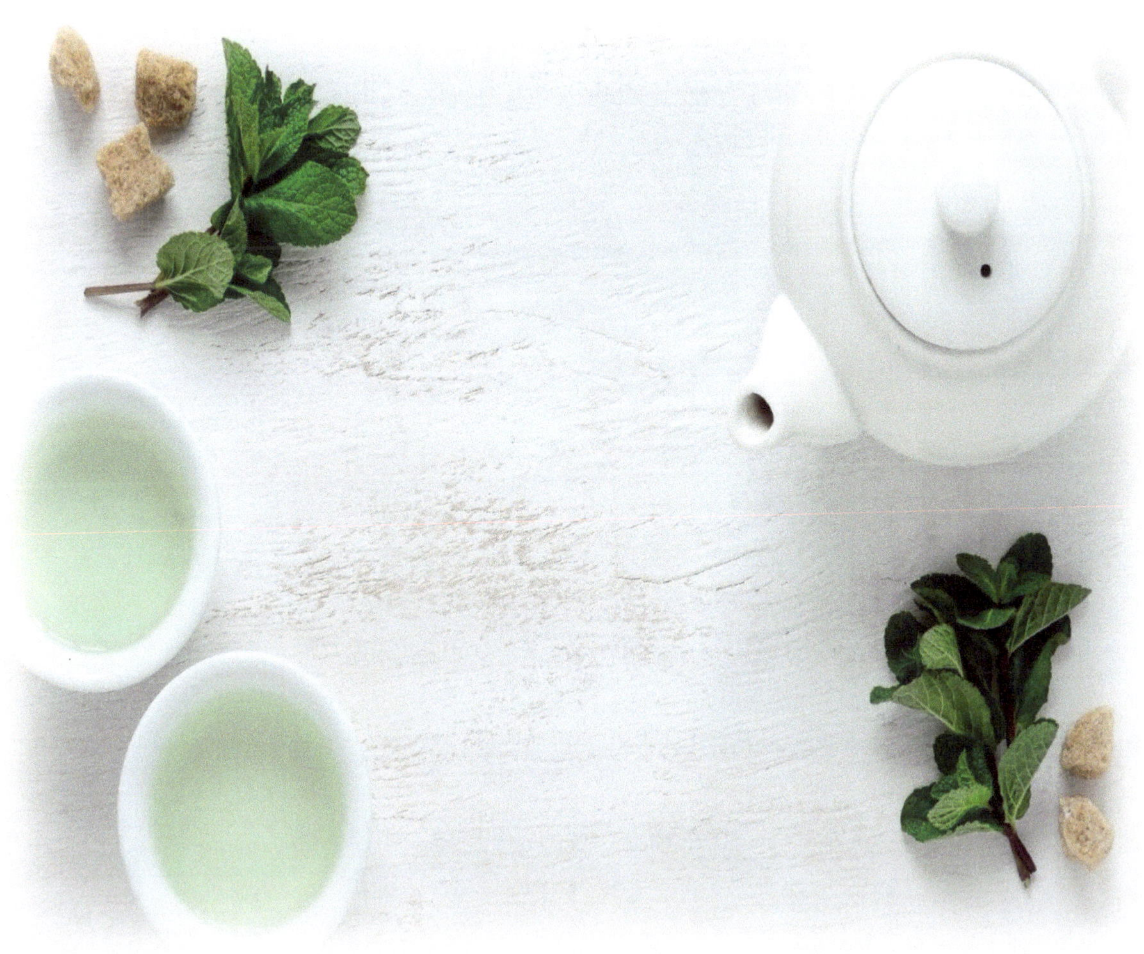

Honey, No More Pimples!

Naturally dries out stubborn, hard to manage acne.

Ingredients:

- 1 Tbsp. Honey

- 1 tsp. Cinnamon

Instructions:

Microwave ingredients together until desired warmth. Stir thoroughly. Apply generously on stubborn pimples. Allow 12-15 minutes for mixture to dry all the way. Rinse with warm water, and pat dry with clean towel. *****Do not apply this mixture all over face, or on clear skin. It is intended for troubling pimples only*****

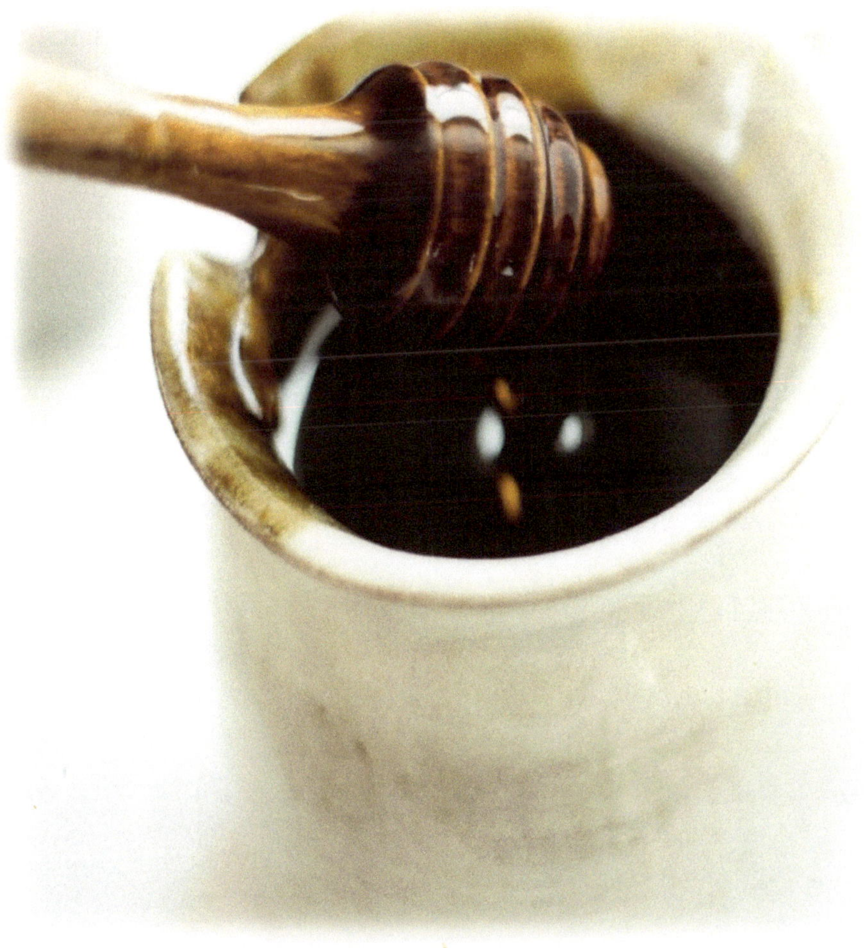

Cocoa Glow

Great for all skin types! Cleanses, hydrates, and leaves skin beaming with a. naturally beautiful glow.

Ingredients:

- 2 Tbsp. Plain Yogurt

- 1 tsp. Cocoa Powder

- 1 Tbsp. Honey

Instructions:

Warm honey in microwave if preferred. Stir honey and cocoa powder together thoroughly, then mix in yogurt. Apply to clean face, and allow 15-20 minutes of time to pass. Don't worry, this mask may not dry completely! Rinse with warm water, pat dry with clean towel.

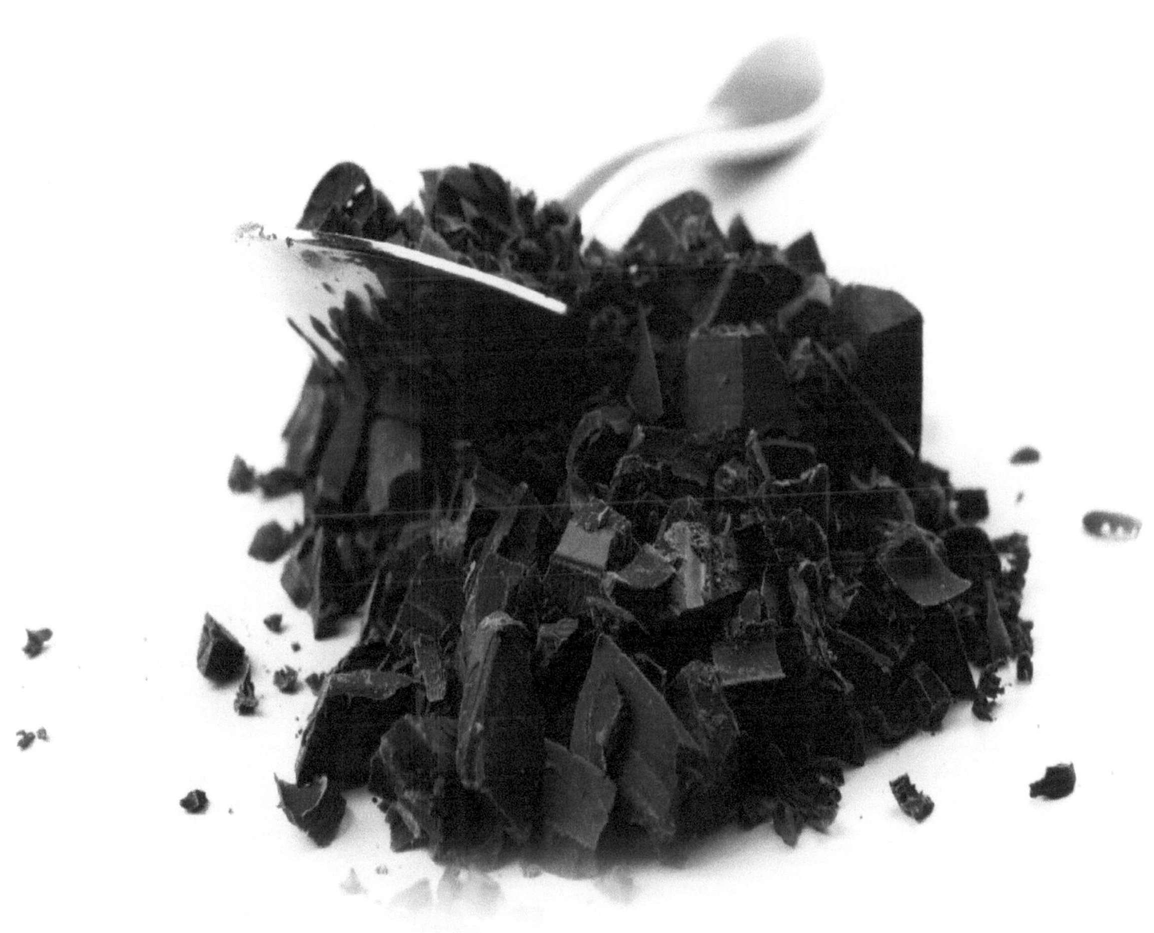

Turmeric Squeeze

Helps tighten loose skin, and reduces the appearance of wrinkles.

Ingredients:

- 1 Tbsp. Turmeric Powder

- 1-2 tsp. Fresh Lemon Juice

- 1 Egg White (preferably organic)

Instructions:

Beat egg white thoroughly. Stir in fresh lemon juice, and turmeric powder until mixture is smooth. Liberally apply to skin, and allow mask to dry for 10-12 minutes. Rinse with warm water, and pat dry with clean towel.

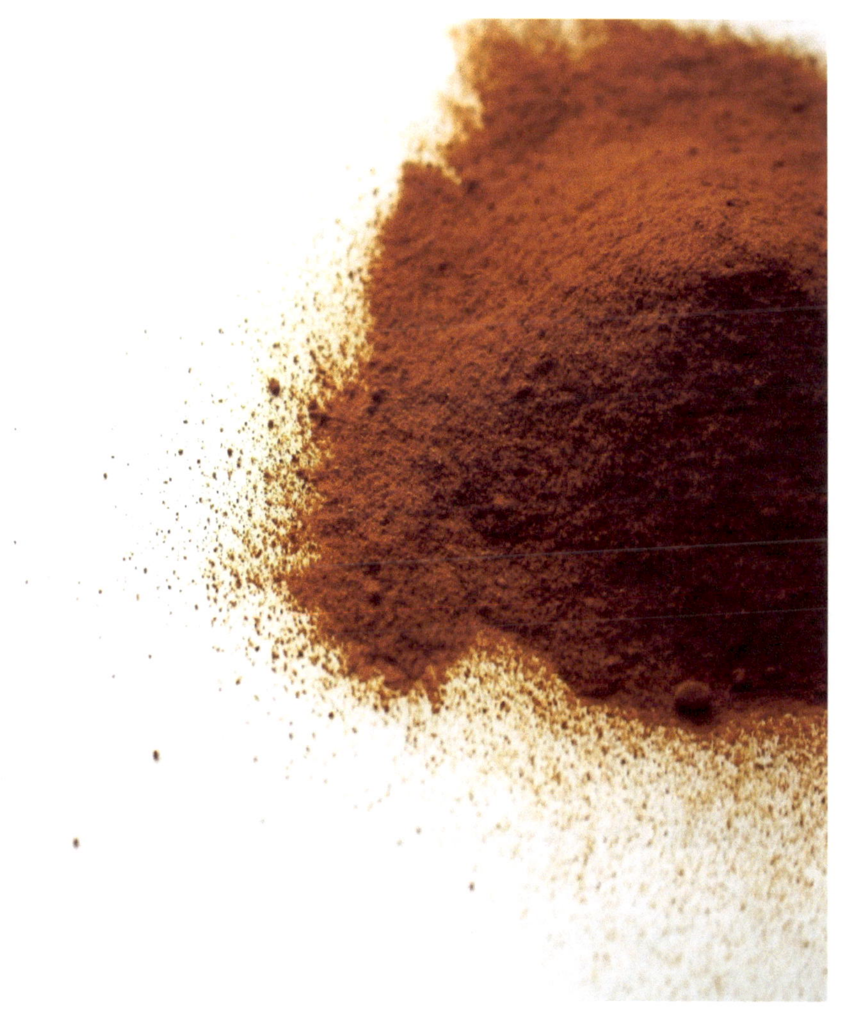

Bare Necessities

A must try for every skin type.

Ingredients:

- 1 Tbsp. Honey

- ½ Cup of Milk, or Almond Milk

- ½ Cup Oats

- ¼-½ Cup of Water

Instructions:

Cook all ingredients together for 4-5 minutes in a sauce pan. Medium heat

works best. Massage mask into skin, and relax for 15-20 minutes. Rinse with

warm water, and pat dry with clean towel.

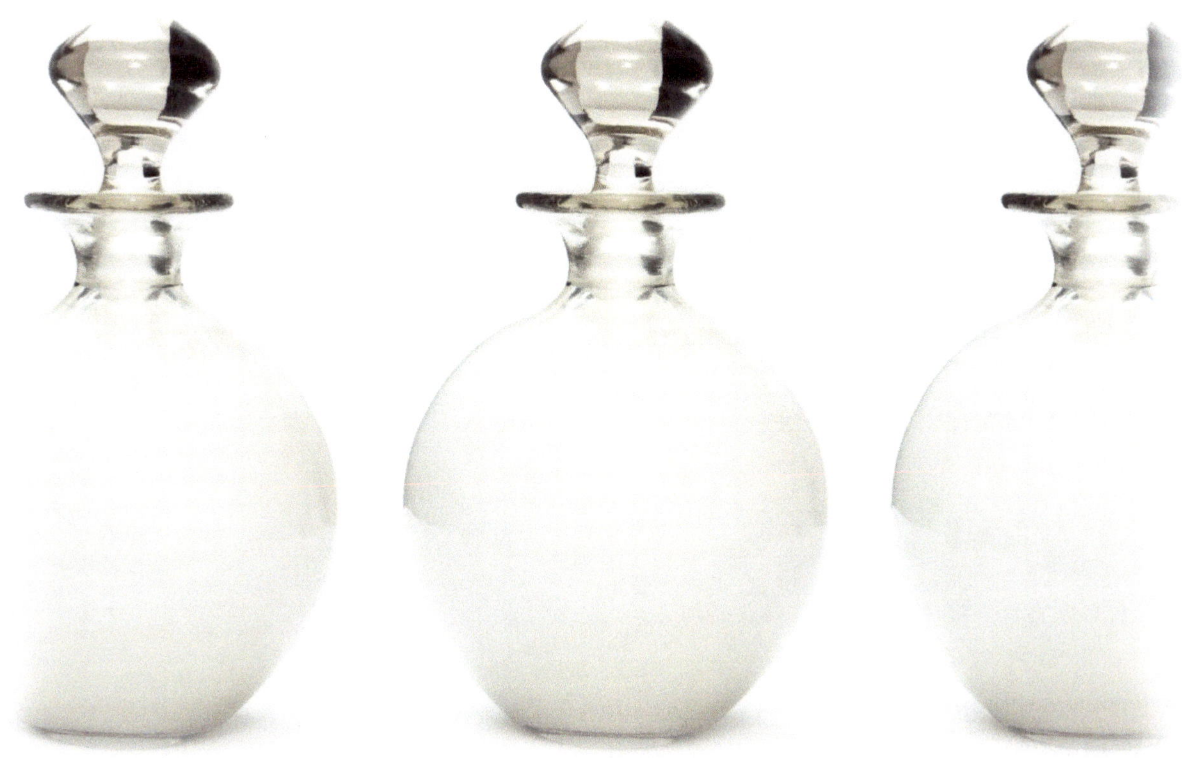

Caffeinated and Bright

Reverses aging skin, reduces sun damage, protects against free radicals, and naturally illuminates skin.

Ingredients:

- 1 Tbsp. Coffee Grounds

- 1 Tbsp. Cocoa Powder

- 1 tsp. Honey

- 1-2 Tbsp. Milk or Almond Milk

Instructions:

Combine coffee grounds and cocoa powder. Add honey and milk. Stir vigorously. Depending on desired thickness of mask, add more or less milk until anticipated texture is achieved. Scrub mask onto skin, and allow 12-15 minutes to pass. Rinse with warm water, and pat dry with clean towel.

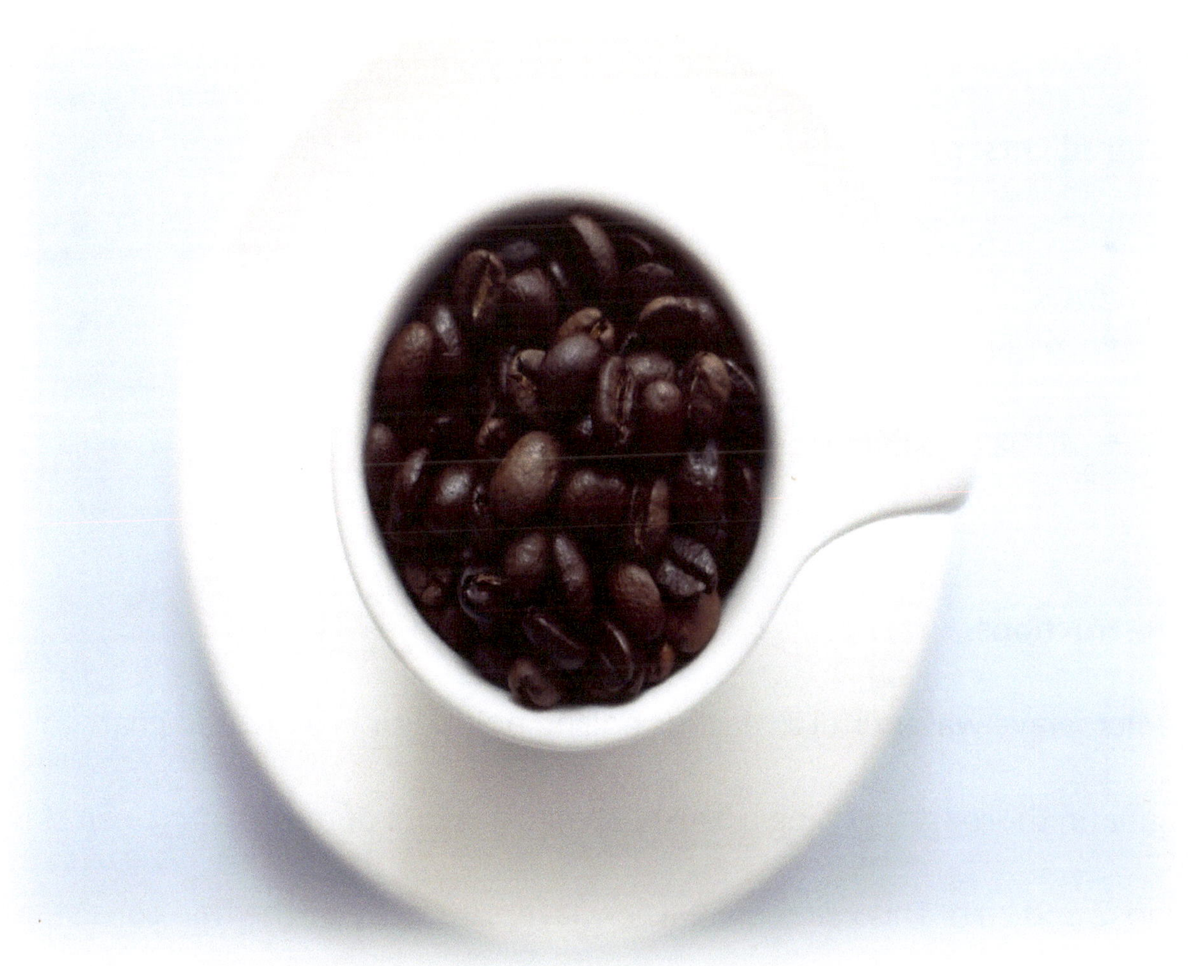

Charcoal Peel

Pull blackheads directly out of your skin!

Ingredients: p

- ½ tsp. Activated Charcoal

- ½ tsp. Unflavored Gelatin

- 1 Tbsp. Water

Instructions:

Microwave water until it reaches boiling point. Stir in activated charcoal, and gelatin thoroughly. Using a brush, paint 2-3 layers of mask onto clean skin on nose and chin. This will require a few layers because of the thin consistency. Place a small strip of paper towel <u>over the first 2-3 layers of mask</u>. Paint 2-3 more layers <u>on top of the paper towel strips</u>. This will prevent the mask from cracking and falling off before we are ready to peel. **Avoid putting this mask on or near eyebrows, it will pull them off. I recommend only using this on your nose and chin.** This mask requires roughly 40-45 minutes to dry before it is time to peel. When mask is completely dry, it will become very hard. If consistency is rubbery or soft, allow more time to dry for full effect. Peel mask off gently, and slowly. It can be painful if you are not careful. Skin may have some redness after removing mask. Rinse face with warm water, pat dry with clean towel,and apply your favorite facial moisturizer.

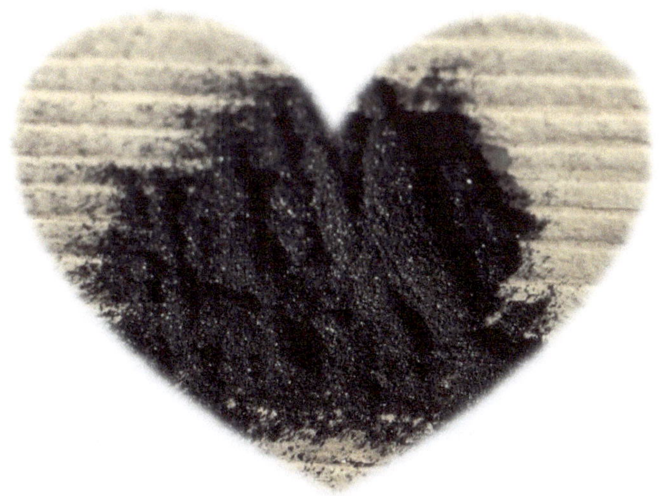

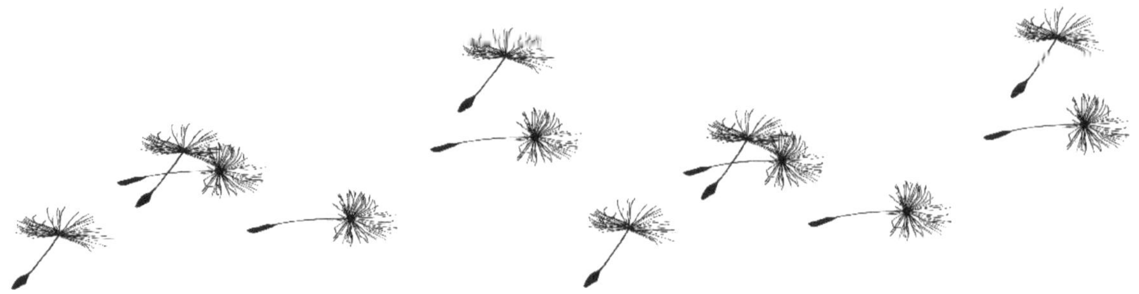

I hope you enjoyed these recipes as much as I did perfecting them in my kitchen! Spoonful of Happy will be releasing full versions of our recipe books in the near future. We look forward to sharing them with you! Until then, check out our website www.spoonfulofhappy.org.

Hashtag your Facebook and Instagram photos showcasing the recipes you recreate **#SpoonfulofHappy**, and follow **@spoonful.of.happy** for a chance to win free products and services! If you have any comment, concerns, or feedback you are welcome to email Spoonful of Happy at **myspoonfulofhappy@gmail.com.**

Kindness looks beautiful on you.

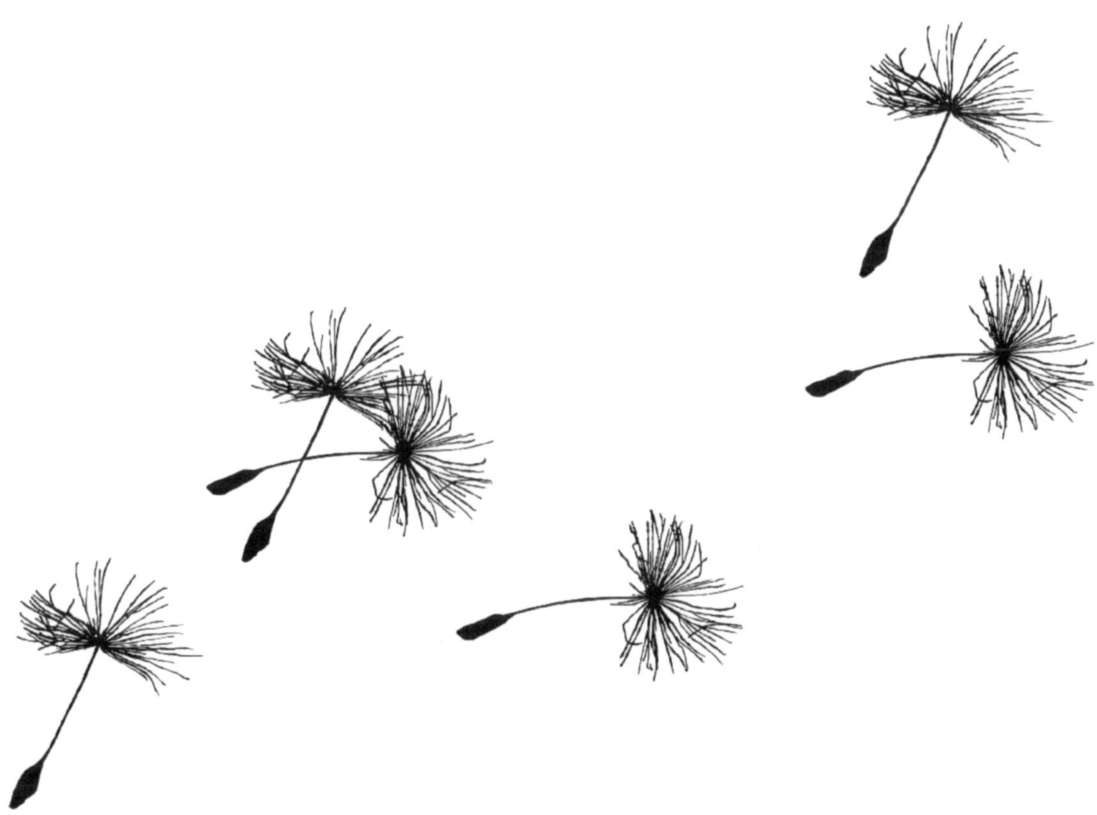

What is Spoonful of Happy?

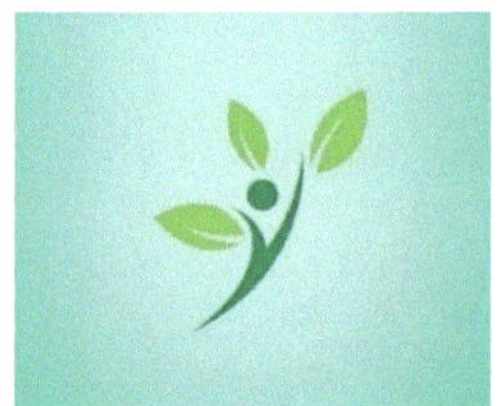

You are probably wondering who I am, and exactly what you can expect from Spoonful of Happy in the future. My name is Makenzee and I am from Boise, Idaho. I have chosen to earn my bachelor's degree in Holistic Nutrition and pursue a career dedicated to health and wellness. I will be accepting one-on-one clients who feel their life can benefit from making dietary and supplemental changes. Multiple packages will be available and I will be accommodating for online, long-distance clients as well. My desire to become a nutritionist was discovered through my own personal health issues and experiences. In 2015 I went from overweight, to underweight, to competing in NPC fitness bikini competitions in only six months. Developing an eating disorder took away my happiness and passion for life quickly. After reaching out for help and receiving the support I needed, I was capable of recovering from my eating disorder. However, just because I am in recovery does not mean I don't struggle. I am human, and the lifelong struggle comes with having an eating disorder. The medical professionals who provided me with the tools I needed to take my life back are appreciated so much, and I cannot express enough gratitude for what they have done for me. But my recovery was lonely and isolating when it did not have to be. I felt like I was the only person in the world who was suffering through an eating disorder. Nobody told me there are **70 MILLION** other people worldwide suffering with something very similar to what I was. Spoonful of Happy is here to break this stigma, and show the world eating disorders are nothing to be ashamed of. These conversations need to be happening and men and women need to feel capable of opening up about their struggles when it comes to food and body image.

Having an eating disorder for so many years also triggered an autoimmune disease. I have been diagnosed by one doctor with celiac disease, and I am in the process of receiving a second opinion to validate exactly what my body is going through. I have chosen to live a gluten-free lifestyle in order to accommodate my disease and prevent damaging my digestive system.

 Going through the eating disorder recovery process and now managing an autoimmune disease has been far from easy. But I can say with confidence that being nutritionally balanced again saved my life. My education along with my personal experiences gives me confidence in my career choice. I am beyond ecstatic to assist others with these very important lifestyle changes!

For more information on exactly what to expect from me and my business in the future, please visit:

www.spoonfulofhappy.org

Feel free to email me at myspoonfulofhappy@gmail.com.

If you or someone you love are suffering from an eating disorder and need help, the National Eating Disorder Hotline is:

1-800-931-2237

Would you benefit from hiring a nutritionist?

Y/ N I struggle to wake up in the morning without consuming caffeine.

Y/N My periods are irregular, painful, and out of control.

Y/N I have an autoimmune disease, chronic illness, and/or take prescription medications.

Y/N I am prone to infection and seem to catch every "bug" going around.

Y/N I feel the urge to urinate frequently, have chronic UTIs, and burning in my urethra when relieving myself.

Y/N Sex is painful, causes bleeding, or does not exist due to no sex drive.

Y/N Sugar cravings happen often, and it is difficult to say no to sweet treats.

Y/N I eat out at least three times a week.

Y/N It is difficult to have water with my meals instead of a soft drink, juice, or milk.

Y/N My lack of energy throughout the day effects my performance at home, work, and/or school.

Y/N I have been diagnosed with a form of ADHD, depression, anxiety, or personality disorder.

Y/N I obsess about my weight and/or body fat percentage.

Y/N My health decisions have an impact on the people I love around me.

Y/N I am in charge of meal planning for my family.

Y/N My bowel movements are irregular, and diarrhea and/or constipation cause me discomfort, and interrupt my daily schedule often.

Y/N My skin is sensitive to light, and I sunburn/get blisters easily.

Y/N My skin is prone to breaking out in eczema, hives, and/or psoriasis.

Y/N I get acne on my face, shoulders, back, buttocks, and/or chest and can't seem to get it under control.

Y/N My hair is thinning, scalp gets scaly/itchy, and does not seem to grow well.

Y/N My fingernails are dry, brittle, and crack easily.

Y/N The weather tends to play a major role in my mood.

Y/N Meal prepping seems tedious, and I would rather skip lunch or grab something convenient.

Y/N I prepare my children and/or spouse's meals.

Y/N My weight fluctuates drastically due to my poor diet.

Y/N I get cold sores, fever blisters, receding gum lines, or open canker sores in my mouth and I usually do not know what triggers them.

Y/N I am uncomfortable in my own skin, and tend to compare my body and lifestyle to others around me.

Y/N 40% or more of food at home consists of processed foods in boxes/packages.

Y/N I do not see the value in eating cage free eggs, organic veggies/fruit, and grass fed meat when it is so expensive.

Y/N I feel the need to purge or restrict calories.

Y/N When I eat, sometimes I find it hard to stop when I am full.

Y/N I have participated in a crash diet, or purchased a workout program/trainer that promised results I did not receive.

Y/N I have the desire to make lifestyle changes! I want my life to be more fulfilling, and reap the benefits of living a healthy life.

If you answered YES to ANY of the questions above, you would absolutely benefit from hiring a personal nutritionist to assist you, and/or your family with important lifestyle changes.

At Spoonful of Happy, we are dedicated to integrating a new healthy lifestyle in a realistic way that is fail proof. Our mission will always keep our client's best interest in mind. Checkout our individual, and family packages on our website www.spoonfulofhappy.org , or email us at myspoonfulofhappy@gmail.com if you have any questions or concerns.

XO. –Spoonful of Happy.

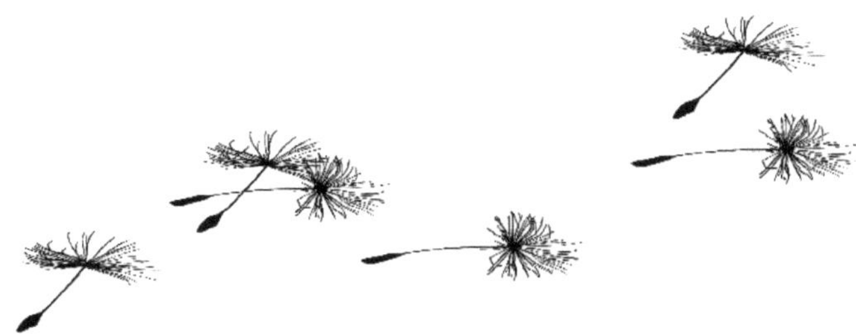

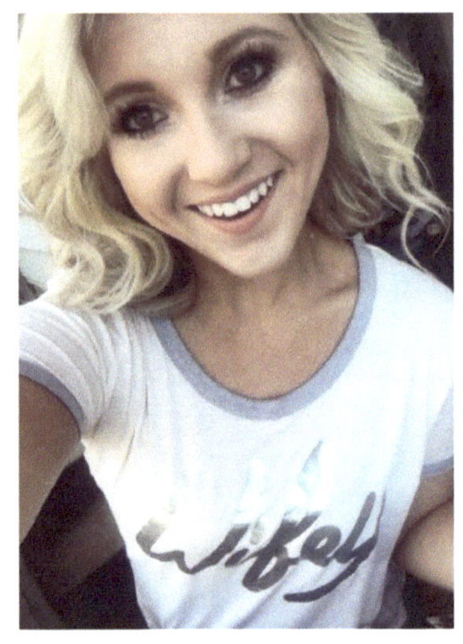

- Founder of Spoonful of Happy.

- Holistic Nutritional Therapy Practitioner.

- Published Author/Blogger/Vlogger.

- Eating Disorder Survivor.

- Healthy Lifestyle Promoter.

- Specialized Nutrition Research Expert.

- Recipe Creator.

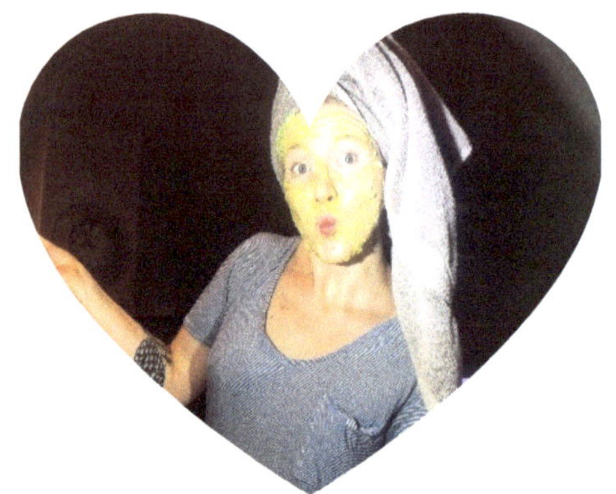

Makenzee Peterson